Plant Based Coo
Beginne

Delicious and Healthy Plant-Based Recipes to Boost your Health

Anna Blank

from various sources. Please consult a licensed professional before attempting any techniques outlined in this book.

By reading this document, the reader agrees that under no circumstances is the author responsible for any losses, direct or indirect, which are incurred as a result of the use of information contained within this document, including, but not limited to, — errors, omissions, or inaccuracies.

Table of Contents

Dark Chocolate Quinoa Breakfast Bowl

- Preparation Time: 15-30 minutes | Cooking Time: 30 minutes | Servings: 4

Ingredients:

- Uncooked white quinoa: 1 cup
- Unsweetened almond milk: 1 cup
- Coconut milk: 1 cup
- Sea salt: 1 pinch
- Unsweetened cocoa powder: 2 tbsp
- Maple syrup: 2-3 tbsp
- Pure vanilla extract: 1/2 tsp
- Vegan dark chocolate: 3-4 squares

Directions:

- Rinse quinoa in a strainer
- Heat the pan and add rinsed quinoa and dry them up
- Add coconut milk, almond milk, and salt
- Lower the heat to medium and stir gently for 20 minutes
- Remove from heat after quinoa is tender
- Add vanilla and maple syrup and serve

Nutrition:

- Carbs: 40. 9 Protein: 7. 5g Fats: 6. 7g Calories: 236 Kcal

Quinoa Black Beans Breakfast Bowl

• Preparation Time: 5-15 minutes | Cooking Time: 25 minutes | Servings: 4

Ingredients:

- 1 cup brown quinoa, rinsed well
- Salt to taste
- 3 tbsp plant-based yogurt
- ½ lime, juiced
- 2 tbsp chopped fresh cilantro
- 1 (5 oz) can black beans, drained and rinsed
- 3 tbsp tomato salsa
- ¼ small avocado, pitted, peeled, and sliced
- 2 radishes, shredded
- 1 tbsp pepitas (pumpkin seeds)

Directions:

• Cook the quinoa with 2 cups of slightly salted water in a medium pot over medium heat or until the liquid absorbs, 15 minutes.

• Spoon the quinoa into serving bowls and fluff with a fork.

• In a small bowl, mix the yogurt, lime juice, cilantro,

and salt. Divide this mixture on the quinoa and top with the beans, salsa, avocado, radishes, and pepitas.

- Serve immediately.

Nutrition:

- Calories 131 Fats 3. 5g Carbs 20 Protein 6. 5g

Corn Griddle Cakes With Tofu Mayonnaise

• Preparation Time: 5-15 minutes | Cooking Time: 35 minutes | Servings: 4

Ingredients:

- 1 tbsp flax seed powder + 3 tbsp water
- 1 cup water or as needed
- 2 cups yellow cornmeal
- 1 tsp salt
- 2 tsp baking powder
- 4 tbsp olive oil for frying
- 1 cup tofu mayonnaise for serving

Directions:

• In a medium bowl, mix the flax seed powder with water and allow thickening for 5 minutes to form the flax egg.

• Mix in the water and then whisk in the cornmeal, salt, and baking powder until soup texture forms but not watery.

• Heat a quarter of the olive oil in a griddle pan and pour in a quarter of the batter. Cook until set and golden brown beneath, 3 minutes. Flip the cake and cook the other side until set and golden brown too.

• Plate the cake and make three more with the remaining oil and batter.

• Top the cakes with some tofu mayonnaise before serving.

Nutrition:

• Calories 896 Fats 50. 7g Carbs 91. 6g Protein 17. 3g

Savory Breakfast Salad

• Preparation Time: 15-30 minutes | Cooking Time: 20 minutes | Servings: 2

Ingredients:

- For the sweet potatoes:
- Sweet potato: 2 small
- Salt and pepper: 1 pinch
- Coconut oil: 1 tbsp
- For the Dressing:
- Lemon juice: 3 tbsp
- Salt and pepper: 1 pinch each
- Extra virgin olive oil: 1 tbsp
- For the Salad: Mixed greens: 4 cups
- For Servings: Hummus: 4 tbsp
- Blueberries: 1 cup
- Ripe avocado: 1 medium
- Fresh chopped parsley
- Hemp seeds: 2 tbsp

Directions:

- Take a large skillet and apply gentle heat
- Add sweet potatoes, coat them with salt and pepper and pour some oil
- Cook till sweet potatoes turns browns

- Take a bowl and mix lemon juice, salt, and pepper
- Add salad, sweet potatoes, and the serving together
- Mix well and dress and serve

Nutrition:

- Carbs: 57. 6g Protein: 7. 5g Fats: 37. 6g Calories: 523 Kcal

Almond Plum Oats Overnight

• Preparation Time: 15-30 minutes | Cooking Time: 10 minutes plus overnight | Servings: 2

Ingredients:

- Rolled oats: 60g
- Plums: 3 ripe and chopped
- Almond milk: 300ml
- Chia seeds: 1 tbsp
- Nutmeg: a pinch
- Vanilla extract: a few drops
- Whole almonds: 1 tbsp roughly chopped

Directions:

• Add oats, nutmeg, vanilla extract, almond milk, and chia seeds to a bowl and mix well • Add in cubed plums and cover and place in the fridge for a night

• Mix the oats well next morning and add into the serving bowl

• Serve with your favorite toppings

Nutrition:

• Carbs: 24. 7g Protein: 9. 5g Fats: 10. 8g Calories: 248Kcal

High Protein Toast

• Preparation Time: 15-30 minutes | Cooking Time: 15 minutes | Servings: 2

Ingredients:

- White bean: 1 drained and rinsed
- Cashew cream: ½ cup
- Miso paste: 1 ½ tbsp
- Toasted sesame oil: 1 tsp
- Sesame seeds: 1 tbsp
- Spring onion: 1 finely sliced
- Lemon: 1 half for the juice and half wedged to serve
- Rye bread: 4 slices toasted

Directions:

• In a bowl add sesame oil, white beans, miso, cashew cream, and lemon juice and mash using a potato masher
• Make a spread
• Spread it on a toast and top with spring onions and sesame seeds
• Serve with lemon wedges

Nutrition:

- Carbs: 44. 05 g Protein: 14. 05 g Fats: 9. 25 g

Calories: 332 Kcal

Hummus Carrot Sandwich

• Preparation Time: 15-30 minutes | Cooking Time: 25 minutes | Servings: 2

Ingredients:

• Chickpeas: 1 cup can drain and rinsed
• Tomato: 1 small sliced
• Cucumber: 1 sliced
• Avocado: 1 sliced
• Cumin: 1 tsp
• Carrot: 1 cup diced
• Maple syrup: 1 tsp
• Tahini: 3 tbsp
• Garlic: 1 clove
• Lemon: 2 tbsp
• Extra-virgin olive oil: 2 tbsp
• Salt: as per your need
• Bread slices: 4

Directions:

• Add carrot to the boiling hot water and boil for 15 minutes
• Blend boiled carrots, maple syrup, cumin, chickpeas, tahini, olive oil, salt, and garlic together

in a blender

- Add in lemon juice and mix
- Add to the serving bowl and you can refrigerate for
up to 5 days
- In between two bread slices, spread hummus and
place 2-3 slices of cucumber, avocado, and

tomato and serve

Nutrition:

- Carbs: 53. 15 g Protein: 14. 1 g Fats: 27. 5 g
Calories: 490 Kcal

Overnight Oats

- Preparation Time: 15-30 minutes | Cooking Time: 15 minutes plus overnight | Servings: 6 Ingredients:
  - Cinnamon: a pinch
  - Almond milk: 600ml
  - Porridge oats: 320g Maple syrup: 1 tbsp
  - Pumpkin seeds 1 tbsp
  - Chia seeds: 1 tbsp

Directions:
- Add all the ingredients to the bowl and combine well
- Cover the bowl and place it in the fridge overnight
- Pour more milk in the morning Serve with your favorite toppings

Nutrition:
- Carbs: 32. 3 g Protein: 10. 2 g Fats: 12. 7 g Calories: 298 Kcal

Avocado Miso Chickpeas Toast

• Preparation Time: 15-30 minutes | Cooking Time: 15 minutes | Servings: 2

Ingredients:

- Chickpeas: 400g drained and rinsed
- Avocado: 1 medium
- Toasted sesame oil: 1 tsp
- White miso paste: 1 ½ tbsp
- Sesame seeds: 1 tbsp
- Spring onion: 1 finely sliced
- Lemon: 1 half for the juice and half wedged to serve
- Rye bread: 4 slices toasted

Directions:

- In a bowl add sesame oil, chickpeas, miso, and lemon juice and mash using a potato masher • Roughly crushed avocado in another bowl using a fork
- Add the avocado to the chickpeas and make a spread
- Spread it on a toast and top with spring onion and sesame seeds
- Serve with lemon wedges

Nutrition:

- Carbs: 33. 3 g Protein: 14. 6 g Fats: 26. 6 g Calories: 456 Kcal

Banana Malt Bread

• Preparation Time: 15-30 minutes | Cooking Time: 1 hour 20 minutes and Maturing Time | Servings: 12 slices

Ingredients:

• Hot strong black tea: 120ml
• Malt extract: 150g plus extra for brushing Bananas: 2 ripe mashed
• Sultanas: 100g Pitted dates: 120g chopped
• Plain flour: 250g Soft dark brown sugar: 50g Baking powder: 2 tsp

Directions:

• Preheat the oven to 140C
• Line the loaf tin with the baking paper
• Brew tea and include sultanas and dates to it
• Take a small pan and heat the malt extract and gradually add sugar to it
• Stir continuously and let it cook
• In a bowl, add flour, salt, and baking powder and now top with sugar extract, fruits, bananas, and tea
• Mix the batter well and add to the loaf tin

- Bake the mixture for an hour

- Brush the bread with extra malt extract and let it cool down before removing from the tin • When done, wrap in a foil; it can be consumed for a week

Nutrition:

- Carbs: 43. 3 g Protein: 3. 4 g Fats: 0. 3 g Calories: 194 Kcal

Banana Vegan Bread

• Preparation Time: 15-30 minutes | Cooking Time: 1 hour 15 minutes | Servings: 1 loaf

Ingredients:

• Overripe banana:

• 3 large mashed

• All-purpose flour: 200 g Unsweetened non-dairy milk: 50 ml

• White vinegar: ½ tsp

• Ground flaxseed: 10 g Ground cinnamon: ¼ tsp

• Granulated sugar: 140 g Vanilla: ¼ tsp

• Baking powder: ¼ tsp

• Baking soda: ¼ tsp

• Salt: ¼ tsp

• Canola oil: 3 tbsp

• Chopped walnuts: ½ cup

Directions:

• Preheat the oven to 350F and line the loaf pan with parchment paper

• Mash bananas using a fork

• Take a large bowl, and add in mash bananas, canola oil, oat milk, sugar, vinegar, vanilla, and ground flax seed

- Also whisk in baking powder, cinnamon, flour, and salt
- Add batter to the loaf pan and bake for 50 minutes
- Remove from pan and let it sit for 10 minutes
- Slice when completely cooled down

Nutrition:

- Carbs: 40. 3g Protein: 2. 8g Fats: 8. 2g Calories: 240Kcal

Berry Compote Pancakes

- Preparation Time: 15-30 minutes | Cooking Time: 30 minutes | Servings: 2

Ingredients:

- Mixed frozen berries: 200g
- Plain flour: 140 g
- Unsweetened almond milk: 140ml
- Icing sugar: 1 tbsp
- Lemon juice: 1 tbsp
- Baking powder: 2 tsp
- Vanilla extract: a dash
- Salt: a pinch
- Caster sugar: 2 tbsp
- Vegetable oil: ½ tbsp

Directions:

- Take a small pan and add berries, lemon juice, and icing sugar
- Cook the mixture for 10 minutes to give it a saucy texture and set aside • Take a bowl and add caster sugar, flour, baking powder, and salt and mix well • Add in almond milk and vanilla and combine well to make a batter
- Take a non-stick pan, and heat 2 teaspoons oil in it

and spread it over the whole surface • Add ¼ cup of the batter to the pan and cook each side for 3-4 minutes • Serve with compote

Nutrition:

• Carbs: 92 g Protein: 9. 4 g Fats: 5. 2 g Calories: 463 Kcal

Southwest Breakfast Bowl

• Preparation Time: 15-30 minutes | Cooking Time: 15 minutes | Servings: 1

Ingredients:

• Mushrooms: 1 cup sliced
• Chopped cilantro: ½ cup
• Chili powder: 1 tsp
• Red pepper: 1/2 diced
• Zucchini: 1 cup diced
• Green onion: 1/2 cup chopped
• Onion: 1/2 cup
• Vegan sausage: 1 sliced
• Garlic powder: 1 tsp
• Paprika: 1 tsp
• Cumin: 1/2 tsp
• Salt and pepper: as per your taste
• Avocado: for topping

Directions:

• Put everything in a bowl and apply gentle heat until vegetables turn brown • Pour some pepper and salt as you like and serve with your favorite toppings

Nutrition:

- Carbs: 31. 6g Protein: 33. 8g Fats: 12. 2g Calories: 361

Buckwheat Crepes

• Preparation Time: 15-30 minutes | Cooking Time: 25 minutes | Servings: 12

Ingredients:

- Raw buckwheat flour: 1 cup
- Light coconut milk: 1 and 3/4 cups
- Ground cinnamon: 1/8 tsp
- Flaxseeds: 3/4 tbsp
- Melted coconut oil: 1 tbsp
- Sea salt: a pinch
- Any sweetener: as per your taste

Directions:

• Take a bowl and add flaxseed, coconut milk, salt, avocado, and cinnamon • Mix them all well and fold in the flour

• Now take a nonstick pan and pour oil and provide gentle heat

• Add a big spoon of a mixture

• Cook till it appears bubbly, then change side

• Perform the task until all crepes are prepared

• For enhancing the taste, add the sweetener of your liking

Nutrition:

- Carbs: 8g Protein: 1g Fats: 3g Calories: 71Kcal

Chickpeas Spread Sourdough Toast

• Preparation Time: 15-30 minutes | Cooking Time: 15 minutes | Servings: 4

Ingredients:

- Chickpeas: 1 cup rinsed and drained
- Pumpkin puree: 1 cup
- Vegan yogurt: ½ cup
- Salt: as per your need
- Sourdough: 4 slices toasted

Directions:

• In a bowl add chickpeas and pumpkin puree and mash using a potato masher • Add in salt and yogurt and mix

- Spread it on a toast and serve

Nutrition:

- Carbs: 33. 7g Protein: 8. 45g Fats: 2. 5g Calories: 187Kcal

Chickpeas with Harissa

• Preparation Time: 15-30 minutes | Cooking Time: 20 minutes | Servings: 2

Ingredients:

- Chickpeas: 1 cup can rinse and drained well
- Onion: 1 small diced
- Cucumber: 1 cup diced
- Tomato: 1 cup diced
- Salt: as per your taste
- Lemon juice: 2 tbsp
- Harissa: 2 tsp
- Olive oil: 1 tbsp
- Flat-leaf parsley: 2 tbsp chopped

Directions:

• Add lemon juice, harissa, and olive oil in a bowl and whisk

• Take a serving bowl and add onion, cucumber, chickpeas, salt and the sauce you made • Add parsley from the top and serve

Nutrition:

• Carbs: 55. 6 g Protein: 17. 8g Fats: 11. 8g Calories: 398Kcal

Chocolate Chip Pancake

• Preparation Time: 15-30 minutes | Cooking Time: 30 minutes | Servings: 6 pancakes

Ingredients:

- All-purpose flour: 140g Melted coconut oil: 1 tbsp
- Vegan sugar: 2 tbsp
- Warm almond milk: 250ml
- Baking powder: 1 tbsp
- Sea salt: ¼ tsp
- Chocolate chips: 2 tbsp

Directions:

• Combine together flour, salt, and baking powder and add in chocolate chips • Warm almond milk in the microwave and add sugar and coconut oil and mix well

• There should be no lump in the batter

• Combine together now dry ingredients and the wet ingredients

• Add oil to the non-stick pan on medium heat

• Add ¼ cup of the batter to the pan and cook each side for 3-4 minutes • Serve with vegan butter or any topping you like

Nutrition:

- Amount Per 1 Pancake
- Carbs: 29. 4 g Protein: 3. 1 g Fats: 5 g Calories: 167 Kcal

Coconut, Raspberry, and Chocolate Porridge

• Preparation Time: 15-30 minutes | Cooking Time: 20 minutes | Servings: 2

Ingredients:

- Almond milk: 300 ml
- Quinoa: 80 g Coconut water: 100ml
- Raspberries: 100g Cocoa powder: 1 tbsp
- Coconut sugar: 2 tbsp
- Cocoa nibs: 2 tbsp
- Vegan coconut chips: 2 tbsp toasted

Directions:

• Take a small pan and add coconut water, quinoa, coconut sugar, almond milk, and cocoa powder
- Heat the pan for 20 minutes over medium heat
- Stir continuously in between
- Top with cocoa nibs, coconut chips, and raspberries and serve

Nutrition:

- Carbs: 45. 3 g Protein: 10. 3 g Fats: 19. 3 g Calories: 415 Kcal

Toasted Rye with Pumpkin Seed Butter

• Preparation Time: 15-30 minutes | Cooking Time: 25 minutes and the cooling time | Servings: 4

Ingredients:

- Pumpkin seeds: 220g Date nectar: 1 tsp
- Avocado oil: 2 tbsp
- Rye bread: 4 slices toasted

Directions:

• Toast the pumpkin seed on a frying pan on low heat for 5-7 minutes and stir in between • Let them turn golden and remove from pan

• Add to the blender, when they cool down and make fine powder

• Add in avocado oil and salt and then again blend to form a paste

• Add date nectars too and blend

• On the toasted rye, spread one tablespoon of this butter and serve with your favorite toppings

Nutrition:

• Carbs: 3 g Protein: 5 g Fats: 10. 3 g Calories: 127 Kcal

Vegan Breakfast Hash

• Preparation Time: 15-30 minutes | Cooking Time: 25 minutes | Servings: 4

Ingredients:

• Bell Pepper: 1
• Smoked Paprika: ½ tsp
• Potatoes: 3 medium
• Mushrooms: 8 oz
• Yellow Onion: 1
• Zucchini: 1
• Cumin Powder: ½ tsp
• Garlic Powder: ½ tsp
• Salt and Pepper: as per your taste
• Cooking oil: 2 tbsp (optional)

Directions:

• Heat a large pan on medium flame, add oil and put the sliced potatoes • Cook the potatoes till they change color
• Cut the rest of the vegetables and add all the spices
• Cooked till veggies are soften

Nutrition:

- Carbs: 29. 7g Protein: 5. 5g Fats: 10g Calories: 217 Kcal

Vegan Muffins Breakfast Sandwich

• Preparation Time: 15-30 minutes | Cooking Time: 20 minutes | Servings: 2

Ingredients:

- Romesco Sauce: 3-4 tablespoons
- Fresh baby spinach: ½ cup
- Tofu Scramble: 2
- Vegan English muffins: 2
- Avocado: ½ peeled and sliced
- Sliced fresh tomato: 1

Directions:

- In the oven, toast English muffin
- Half the muffin and spread romesco sauce
- Paste spinach to one side, tailed by avocado slices
- Have warm tofu followed by a tomato slice
- Place the other muffin half onto to the preceding one

Nutrition:

- Carbs: 18g Protein: 12g Fats: 14g Calories: 276 Kcal

Almond Waffles With Cranberries

• Preparation Time: 5-15 minutes | Cooking Time: 20 minutes | Servings: 4 Ingredients:

- 2 tbsp flax seed powder + 6 tbsp water
- 2/3 cup almond flour
- 2 ½ tsp baking powder
- A pinch salt
- 1 ½ cups almond milk
- 2 tbsp plant butter
- 1 cup fresh almond butter
- 2 tbsp pure maple syrup
- 1 tsp fresh lemon juice

Directions:

• In a medium bowl, mix the flax seed powder with water and allow soaking for 5 minutes. • Add the almond flour, baking powder, salt, and almond milk. Mix until well combined. • Preheat a waffle iron and brush with some plant butter. Pour in a quarter cup of the batter,

close the iron and cook until the waffles are golden and crisp, 2 to 3 minutes. • Transfer the waffles to a plate and make more waffles using the same process and ingredient

 proportions.

• Meanwhile, in a medium bowl, mix the almond butter with the maple syrup and lemon juice.

 Serve the waffles, spread the top with the almond-lemon mixture, and serve.

Nutrition:

• Calories 533 Fats 53g Carbs 16. 7g Protein 1. 2g

Chickpea Omelet With Spinach And Mushrooms

• Preparation Time: 5-15 minutes | Cooking Time: 25 minutes | Servings: 4

Ingredients:

- 1 cup chickpea flour
- ½ tsp onion powder
- ½ tsp garlic powder
- ¼ tsp white pepper
- ¼ tsp black pepper
- 1/3 cup nutritional yeast
- ½ tsp baking soda
- 1 small green bell pepper, deseeded and chopped
- 3 scallions, chopped
- 1 cup sautéed sliced white button mushrooms
- ½ cup chopped fresh spinach
- 1 cup halved cherry tomatoes for serving
- 1 tbsp fresh parsley leaves

Directions:

• In a medium bowl, mix the chickpea flour, onion powder, garlic powder, white pepper, black pepper, nutritional yeast, and baking soda until well combined.

• Heat a medium skillet over medium heat and add a quarter of the batter. Swirl the pan to spread the batter across the pan. Scatter a quarter each of the bell pepper, scallions, mushrooms, and spinach on top, and cook until the bottom part of the omelet sets and is golden brown, 1 to 2 minutes. Carefully, flip the omelet and cook the other side until set and golden brown.

• Transfer the omelet to a plate and make the remaining omelets using the remaining batter in the same proportions.

• Serve the omelet with the tomatoes and garnish with the parsley leaves. Serve.

Nutrition:

• Calories 147 Fats 1. 8g Carbs 21. 3g Protein 11. 6g

Sweet Coconut Raspberry Pancakes

- Preparation Time: 5-15 minutes | Cooking Time: 25 minutes | Servings: 4

Ingredients:

- 2 tbsp flax seed powder + 6 tbsp water
- ½ cup of coconut milk
- ¼ cup fresh raspberries, mashed
- ½ cup oat flour
- 1 tsp baking soda
- A pinch salt
- 1 tbsp coconut sugar
- 2 tbsp pure date syrup
- ½ tsp cinnamon powder
- 2 tbsp unsweetened coconut flakes
- 2 tsp plant butter
- Fresh raspberries for garnishing

Directions:

- In a medium bowl, mix the flax seed powder with the water and allow thickening for 5 minutes.
- Mix in the coconut milk and raspberries.
- Add the oat flour, baking soda, salt, coconut sugar,

date syrup, and cinnamon powder. Fold in the coconut flakes until well combined.

• Working in batches, melt a quarter of the butter in a non-stick skillet and add ¼ cup of the batter. Cook until set beneath and golden brown, 2 minutes. Flip the pancake and cook on the other side until set and golden brown, 2 minutes. Transfer to a plate and make the remaining pancakes using the rest of the ingredients in the same proportions.

• Garnish the pancakes with some raspberries and serve warm!

Nutrition:

• Calories 412 Fats 28. 3g Carbs 33. 7g Protein 7. 6g

Pumpkin-Pistachio Tea Cake

• Preparation Time: 5-15 minutes | Cooking Time: 70 minutes | Servings: 4

Ingredients:

- 2 tbsp flaxseed powder + 6 tbsp water
- 3 tbsp vegetable oil
- ¾ cup canned unsweetened pumpkin puree
- ½ cup pure corn syrup
- 3 tbsp pure date sugar
- 1 ½ cups whole-wheat flour
- ½ tsp cinnamon powder
- ½ tsp baking powder
- ¼ tsp cloves powder
- ½ tsp allspice powder
- ½ tsp nutmeg powder
- A pinch salt
- 2 tbsp chopped pistachios

Directions:

• Preheat the oven to 350 F and lightly coat an 8 x 4-inch loaf pan with cooking spray. In a medium bowl, mix the flax seed powder with water and allow thickening for 5 minutes to make the flax egg.

• In a bowl, whisk the vegetable oil, pumpkin puree,

corn syrup, date sugar, and flax egg. In another bowl, mix the flour, cinnamon powder, baking powder, cloves powder, allspice powder, nutmeg powder, and salt. Add this mixture to the wet batter and mix until well combined.

• Pour the batter into the loaf pan, sprinkle the pistachios on top, and gently press the nuts onto the batter to stick.

• Bake in the oven for 50 to 55 minutes or until a toothpick inserted into the cake comes out clean. Remove the cake onto a wire rack, allow cooling, slice, and serve.

Nutrition:
• Calories 330 Fats 13. 2g Carbs 50. 1g Protein 7g

Carrot And Chocolate Bread

- Preparation Time: 5-15 minutes | Cooking Time: 75 minutes | Servings: 4

Ingredients:

- For the dry mix:
- 1 ½ cup whole-wheat flour
- ¼ cup almond flour
- ¼ tsp salt
- ¼ tsp cloves powder
- ¼ tsp cayenne pepper
- 1 tbsp cinnamon powder
- ½ tsp nutmeg powder
- ½ tsp baking soda
- 1 ½ tsp baking powder
- For the wet batter:
- 2 tbsp flax seed powder + 6 tbsp water
- ½ cup pure date sugar
- ¼ cup pure maple syrup
- ¾ tsp almond extract
- 1 tbsp grated lemon zest
- ½ cup unsweetened applesauce
- ¼ cup olive oil
- For folding into the batter:

- 4 carrots, shredded
- 3 tbsp unsweetened chocolate chips
- 2/3 cup black raisins

Directions:

- Preheat the oven to 375 F and line an 8x4 loaf tin with baking paper.
- In a large bowl, mix all the flours, salt, cloves powder, cayenne pepper, cinnamon powder,

nutmeg powder, baking soda, and baking powder.
- In another bowl, mix the flaxseed powder, water, and allow thickening for 5 minutes. Mix in the date sugar, maple syrup, almond extract, lemon zest, applesauce, and olive oil. • Combine both mixtures until smooth and fold in the carrots, chocolate chips, and raisins. • Pour the mixture into a loaf pan and bake in the oven until golden brown on top or a toothpick inserted into the bread comes out clean, 45 to 60 minutes.
- Remove from the oven, transfer the bread onto a wire rack to cool, slice, and serve.

Nutrition:

- Calories 524 Fats 15. 8g Carbs 94. 3g Protein 7. 9g

Pineapple French Toasts

• Preparation Time: 5-15 minutes | Cooking Time: 55 minutes | Servings: 4

Ingredients:

- 2 tbsp flax seed powder + 6 tbsp water
- 1 ½ cups unsweetened almond milk
- ½ cup almond flour
- 2 tbsp pure maple syrup + extra for drizzling
- 2 pinches salt
- ½ tbsp cinnamon powder
- ½ tsp fresh lemon zest
- 1 tbsp fresh pineapple juice
- 8 whole-grain bread slices

Directions:

• Preheat the oven to 400 F and lightly grease a roasting rack with olive oil. Set aside.

• In a medium bowl, mix the flax seed powder with water and allow thickening for 5 to 10 minutes.
• Whisk in the almond milk, almond flour, maple syrup, salt, cinnamon powder, lemon zest, and pineapple juice.
• Soak the bread on both sides in the almond milk mixture and allow sitting on a plate for 2 to 3 minutes.

54

• Heat a large skillet over medium heat and place the bread in the pan. Cook until golden brown on the bottom side. Flip the bread and cook further until golden brown on the other side, 4 minutes in total.

• Transfer to a plate, drizzle some maple syrup on top and serve immediately.

Nutrition:

• Calories 294 Fats 4. 7g Carbs 52. 0g Protein 11. 6g

Pimiento Cheese Breakfast Biscuits

• Preparation Time: 5-15 minutes | Cooking Time: 30 minutes | Servings: 4

Ingredients:

- 2 cups whole-wheat flour
- 2 tsp baking powder
- 1 tsp salt
- ½ tsp baking soda
- ½ tsp garlic powder
- ¼ tsp black pepper
- ¼ cup unsalted plant butter, cold and cut into 1/2-inch cubes
- ¾ cup of coconut milk
- 1 cup shredded cashew cheese
- 1 (4 oz) jar chopped pimientos, well-drained
- 1 tbsp melted unsalted plant butter

Directions:

• Preheat the oven to 450 F and line a baking sheet with parchment paper. Set aside. In a medium bowl, mix the flour, baking powder, salt, baking soda, garlic powder, and black pepper. Add the cold butter using a hand mixer until the mixture is the size of small peas.

- Pour in ¾ of the coconut milk and continue whisking. Continue adding the remaining coconut milk, a tablespoonful at a time, until dough forms.
- Mix in the cashew cheese and pimientos. (If the dough is too wet to handle, mix in a little bit more flour until it is manageable). Place the dough on a lightly floured surface and flatten the dough into ½-inch thickness.
- Use a 2 ½inch round cutter to cut out biscuits` pieces from the dough. Gather, re-roll the dough once and continue cutting out biscuits. Arrange the biscuits on the prepared pan and brush the tops with the melted butter. Bake for 12-14 minutes, or until the biscuits are golden brown. Cool and serve.

Nutrition:
- Calories 1009 Fats 71. 8g Carbs 74. 8g Protein 24. 5g

Breakfast Naan Bread With Mango Saffron Jam

• Preparation Time: 5-15 minutes | Cooking Time: 40 minutes | Servings: 4

Ingredients:

- For the naan bread:
- ¾ cup almond flour
- 1 tsp salt + extra for sprinkling
- 1 tsp baking powder
- 1/3 cup olive oil
- 2 cups boiling water
- 2 tbsp plant butter for frying
- For the mango saffron jam:
- 4 cups heaped chopped mangoes
- 1 cup pure maple syrup
- 1 lemon, juiced
- A pinch of saffron powder
- 1 tsp cardamom powder

Directions:

- For the naan bread:
- In a large bowl, mix the almond flour, salt, and baking powder. Mix in the olive oil and

boiling water until smooth, thick batter forms. Allow the dough to rise for 5 minutes. • Form 6 to 8 balls out of the dough, place each on a baking paper and use your hands to
 flatten the dough.
 • Working in batches, melt the plant butter in a large skillet and fry the dough on both sides
 until set and golden brown on each side, 4 minutes per bread. Transfer to a plate and set aside
 for serving.
 • For the mango saffron jam
 • Add the mangoes, maple syrup, lemon juice, and 3 tbsp of water in a medium pot and cook
 over medium heat until boiling, 5 minutes.
 • Mix in the saffron and cardamom powders and cook further over low heat until the mangoes
 are softened.
 • Mash the mangoes with the back of the spoon until fairly smooth with little chunks of
 mangoes in the jam.
 • Turn the heat off and cool completely. Spoon the jam into sterilized jars and serve with the
 naan bread.

Nutrition:

- Calories 766 Fats 42. 7g Carbs 93. 8g Protein 7. 3g

Cauliflower And Potato Hash Browns

- Preparation Time: 5-15 minutes | Cooking Time: 35 minutes | Servings: 4 Ingredients:
- 3 tbsp flax seed powder + 9 tbsp water
- 2 large potatoes, peeled and shredded
- 1 big head cauliflower, rinsed and riced
- ½ white onion, grated
- 1 tsp salt
- 1 tbsp black pepper
- 4 tbsp plant butter, for frying

Directions:

- In a medium bowl, mix the flaxseed powder and water. Allow thickening for 5 minutes for the flax egg.
- Add the potatoes, cauliflower, onion, salt, and black pepper to the flax egg and mix until well combined. Allow sitting for 5 minutes to thicken.
- Working in batches, melt 1 tbsp of plant butter in a non-stick skillet and add 4 scoops of the hash brown mixture to the skillet. Make sure to have 1 to 2-inch intervals between each scoop.
- Use the spoon to flatten the batter and cook until

compacted and golden brown on the bottom part, 2 minutes. Flip the hashbrowns and cook further for 2 minutes or until the vegetables are cooked and golden brown. Transfer to a paper towel-lined plate to drain grease.

• Make the remaining hashbrowns using the remaining ingredients.

• Serve warm.

Nutrition:

• Calories 265 Fats 11. 9g Carbs 36. 7g Protein 5. 3g

Raspberry Raisin Muffins With Orange Glaze

• Preparation Time: 5-15 minutes | Cooking Time: 40 minutes | Servings: 4

Ingredients:

- For the muffins:
- 2 tbsp flax seed powder + 6 tbsp water
- 2 cups whole-wheat flour
- 1½ tsp baking powder
- A pinch salt
- ½ cup plant butter, room temperature
- 1 cup pure date sugar
- ½ cup oat milk
- 2 tsp vanilla extract
- 1 lemon, zested
- 1 cup dried raspberries
- For the orange glaze:
- 2 tbsp orange juice
- 1 cup pure date sugar

Directions:

• Preheat the oven to 400 F and grease 6 muffin cups with cooking spray. In a small bowl, mix the flax seed powder with water and allow thickening for 5 minutes to make the flax egg. In a medium bowl, mix the flour, baking powder, and salt. In another bowl, cream the plant butter, date sugar, and flax egg. Mix in the oat milk, vanilla, and lemon zest.

• Combine both mixtures, fold in raspberries, and fill muffin cups two-thirds way up with the batter. Bake until a toothpick inserted comes out clean, 20-25 minutes.

• In a medium bowl, whisk orange juice and date sugar until smooth. Remove the muffins when ready and transfer them to a wire rack to cool. Drizzle the glaze on top to serve.

Nutrition:
• Calories 700 Fats 25. 5g Carbs 115. 1g Protein 10. 5g

Berry Cream Compote Over Crepes

• Preparation Time: 5-15 minutes | Cooking Time: 35 minutes | Servings: 4

Ingredients:

- • For the berry cream:
- 1 knob plant butter
- 2 tbsp pure date sugar
- 1 tsp vanilla extract
- ½ cup fresh blueberries
- ½ cup fresh raspberries
- ½ cup whipped coconut cream
- For the crepes:
- 2 tbsp flax seed powder + 6 tbsp water
- 1 tsp vanilla extract
- 1 tsp pure date sugar
- ¼ tsp salt
- 2 cups almond flour
- 1 ½ cups almond milk
- 1 ½ cups water
- 3 tbsp plant butter for frying

Directions:

• Melt butter in a pot over low heat and mix in the date sugar, and vanilla. Cook until the sugar melts and then toss in berries. Allow softening for 2 3 minutes. Set aside to cool.

• In a medium bowl, mix the flax seed powder with water and allow thickening for 5 minutes to make the flax egg. Whisk in the vanilla, date sugar, and salt.

• Pour in a quarter cup of almond flour and whisk, then a quarter cup of almond milk, and mix until no lumps remain. Repeat the mixing process with the remaining almond flour and almond milk in the same quantities until exhausted.

• Mix in 1 cup of water until the mixture is runny like that of pancakes and add the remaining water until the mixture is lighter. Brush a large non-stick skillet with some butter and place over medium heat to melt.

• Pour 1 tablespoon of the batter into the pan and swirl the skillet quickly and all around to coat the pan with the batter. Cook until the batter is dry and golden brown beneath, about 30 seconds.

• Use a spatula to carefully flip the crepe and cook the other side until golden brown too. Fold the crepe onto a plate and set aside. Repeat making more crepes with the remaining batter until exhausted. Plate the crepes, top with the whipped coconut cream, and the berry compote. Serve immediately.

Nutrition:

- Calories 339 Fats 24. 5g Carbs 30g Protein 2. 3g

Irish Brown Bread

• Preparation Time: 5-15 minutes | Cooking Time: 50 minutes | Servings: 4

Ingredients:
- 4 cups whole-wheat flour
- ¼ tsp salt
- ½ cup rolled oats
- 1 tsp baking soda
- 1 ¾ cups coconut milk, thick
- 2 tbsp pure maple syrup

Directions:
- Preheat the oven to 400 F.
- In a bowl, mix flour, salt, oats, and baking soda. Add in coconut milk, maple syrup, and

whisk until dough forms. Dust your hands with some flour and knead the dough into a ball. Shape the dough into a circle and place on a baking sheet.

• Cut a deep cross on the dough and bake in the oven for 15 minutes at 450 F. Then, reduce the temperature to 400 F and bake further for 20 to 25 minutes or until a hollow sound is made when the bottom of the bread is tapped. Slice and serve.

Nutrition:

- Calories 963 Fats 44. 4g Carbs 125. 1g Protein 22. 1g

Apple Cinnamon Muffins

• Preparation Time: 5-15 minutes | Cooking Time: 40 minutes | Servings: 4

Ingredients:

- For the muffins:
- 1 flax seed powder + 3 tbsp water
- 1 ½ cups whole-wheat flour
- ¾ cup pure date sugar
- 2 tsp baking powder
- ¼ tsp salt
- 1 tsp cinnamon powder
- 1/3 cup melted plant butter
- 1/3 cup flax milk
- 2 apples, peeled, cored, and chopped
- For topping:
- 1/3 cup whole-wheat flour
- ½ cup pure date sugar
- ½ cup cold plant butter, cubed
- 1 ½ tsp cinnamon powder

Directions:

• Preheat the oven to 400 F and grease 6 muffin cups with cooking spray. In a bowl, mix the flax seed powder

70

with water and allow thickening for 5 minutes to make the flax egg.

• In a medium bowl, mix the flour, date sugar, baking powder, salt, and cinnamon powder. Whisk in the butter, flax egg, flax milk, and then fold in the apples. Fill the muffin cups twothirds way up with the batter.

• In a small bowl, mix the remaining flour, date sugar, cold butter, and cinnamon powder. Sprinkle the mixture on the muffin batter. Bake for 20-minutes. Remove the muffins onto a wire rack, allow cooling, and serve warm.

Nutrition:
• Calories 1133 Fats 74. 9g Carbs 104. 3g Protein 18g

Mixed Berry Walnut Yogurt

• Preparation Time: 5-15 minutes | Cooking Time: 10 minutes | Servings: 4

Ingredients:

- 4 cups almond milk Dairy-Free yogurt, cold
- 2 tbsp pure malt syrup
- 2 cups mixed berries, halved or chopped
- ¼ cup chopped toasted walnuts

Directions:

• In a medium bowl, mix the yogurt and malt syrup until well-combined. Divide the mixture into 4 breakfast bowls.
- Top with the berries and walnuts.
- Enjoy immediately.

Nutrition:

- Calories 326 Fats 14. 3g Carbs 38. 3g Protein 12. 5g

Orange Butter Crepes

• Preparation Time: 5-15 minutes | Cooking Time: 30 minutes | Servings: 4

- 2 tbsp flax seed powder + 6 tbsp water
- 1 tsp vanilla extract
- 1 tsp pure date sugar
- ¼ tsp salt
- 2 cups almond flour
- 1½ cups oat milk
- ½ cup melted plant butter
- 3 tbsp fresh orange juice
- 3 tbsp plant butter for frying

Directions:

• In a medium bowl, mix the flax seed powder with 1 cup water and allow thickening for 5 minutes to make the flax egg. Whisk in the vanilla, date sugar, and salt.

• Pour in a quarter cup of almond flour and whisk, then a quarter cup of oat milk, and mix until no lumps remain. Repeat the mixing process with the remaining almond flour and almond milk in the same quantities until exhausted.

• Mix in the plant butter, orange juice, and half of the

water until the mixture is runny like that of pancakes. Add the remaining water until the mixture is lighter. Brush a large non-stick skillet with some butter and place over medium heat to melt.

• Pour 1 tablespoon of the batter into the pan and swirl the skillet quickly and all around to coat the pan with the batter. Cook until the batter is dry and golden brown beneath, about 30 seconds.

• Use a spatula to carefully flip the crepe and cook the other side until golden brown too. Fold the crepe onto a plate and set aside. Repeat making more crepes with the remaining batter until exhausted. Drizzle some maple syrup on the crepes and serve.

Nutrition:

• Calories 379 Fats 35. 6g Carbs 14. 8g Protein 5. 6g

Creole Tofu Scramble

• Preparation Time: 5-15 minutes | Cooking Time: 20 minutes | Servings: 4

Ingredients:

- 2 tbsp plant butter, for frying
- 1 (14 oz) pack firm tofu, pressed and crumbled
- 1 medium red bell pepper, deseeded and chopped
- 1 medium green bell pepper, deseeded and chopped
- 1 tomato, finely chopped
- 2 tbsp chopped fresh green onions
- Salt and black pepper to taste
- 1 tsp turmeric powder
- 1 tsp Creole seasoning
- ½ cup chopped baby kale
- ¼ cup grated plant-based Parmesan cheese

Directions:

• Melt the plant butter in a large skillet over medium heat and add the tofu. Cook with occasional stirring until the tofu is light golden brown while making sure not to break the tofu into tiny bits but to have scrambled egg resemblance, 5 minutes.

• Stir in the bell peppers, tomato, green onions, salt, black pepper, turmeric powder, and Creole seasoning. Sauté until the vegetables soften, 5 minutes.

• Mix in the kale to wilt, 3 minutes and then, half of the plant-based Parmesan cheese. Allow melting for 1 to 2 minutes and then turn the heat off.

• Dish the food, top with the remaining cheese, and serve warm.

Nutrition:

• Calories 258 Fats 15. 9g Carbs 12. 8g Protein 20. 7g

Mushroom Avocado Panini

• Preparation Time: 5-15 minutes | Cooking Time: 30 minutes | Servings: 4

Ingredients:

- 1 tbsp olive oil
- 1 cup sliced white button mushrooms
- Salt and black pepper to taste
- 1 ripe avocado, pitted, peeled, and sliced
- 2 tbsp freshly squeezed lemon juice
- 1 tbsp chopped parsley
- ½ tsp pure maple syrup
- 8 slices whole-wheat ciabatta
- 4 oz sliced plant-based Parmesan cheese
- 1 tbsp olive oil

Directions:

• Heat the olive oil in a medium skillet over medium heat and sauté the mushrooms until softened, 5 minutes. Season with salt and black pepper. Turn the heat off.

• Preheat a panini press to medium heat, 3 to 5 minutes.

• Mash the avocado in a medium bowl and mix in the

lemon juice, parsley, and maple syrup.

• Spread the mixture on 4 bread slices, divide the mushrooms and plant-based Parmesan cheese on top.

• Cover with the other bread slices and brush the top with olive oil.

• Grill the sandwiches one after another in the heated press until golden brown and the cheese melted.

• Serve warm.

Nutrition:

• Calories 338 Fats 22. 4g Carbs 25. 5g Protein 12. 4g

Avocado Toast with Herbs and Peas

Preparation Time: 10 minutes | Cooking Time: 0 minute | Servings: 4

- ½ of a medium avocado, peeled, pitted, mashed
- 6 slices of radish
- 2 tablespoons baby peas
- ¼ teaspoon ground black pepper
- 1 teaspoon chopped basil
- ¼ teaspoon salt
- 1/2 lemon, juiced
- 1 slice of bread, whole-grain, toasted

Directions:

- Spread mashed avocado on one side of the toast and then top with peas, pressing them into the avocado.
- Layer the toast with radish slices, season with salt and black pepper, sprinkle with basil and drizzle with lemon juice.
- Serve straight away.

Nutrition:

- Calories: 250 Cal Fat: 12 g Carbs: 22 g Protein: 7 g Fiber: 9 g

Small Sweet Potato Pancakes

Preparation Time: 20 minutes | Cooking Time: 0 minutes | Servings: 2

Ingredients:

- 1 clove of garlic
- 3 tablespoon wholemeal rice flour
- 1 pinch of nutmeg
- 3 tablespoons of water
- 150 g sweet potato
- 1 pinch of chili flakes
- 1 teaspoon oil
- Salt

Directions:

- Peel the garlic clove and mash it with a fork. Peel the sweet potato and grate it into small sticks with a grater.
- Knead the sweet potato and garlic in a bowl with the rice flour and water, then season with chili flakes, salt, and nutmeg.
- Heat the oil in a pan and form small buffers.
- Fry these in the pan on both sides until golden brown.
- Goes perfectly with tzatziki and other fresh dips.

Nutrition:

• Calories: 209 Fat: 15.4g Carbs: 10.5g Protein: 8.1g
Fiber: 3.2g

Tomato and Pesto Toast

Preparation Time: 5 minutes | Cooking Time: 0 minute | Servings: 4

Ingredients:

- 1 small tomato, sliced
- ¼ teaspoon ground black pepper
- 1 tablespoon vegan pesto
- 2 tablespoons hummus
- 1 slice of whole-grain bread, toasted
- Hemp seeds as needed for garnishing

Directions:

• Spread hummus on one side of the toast, top with tomato slices and then drizzle with pesto. • Sprinkle black pepper on the toast along with hemp seeds and then serve straight away.

Nutrition:

• Calories: 214 Cal Fat: 7.2 g Carbs: 32 g Protein: 6.5 g Fiber: 3 g

Avocado and Sprout Toast

Preparation Time: 5 minutes | Cooking Time: 0 minute |
Servings: 4

Ingredients:

- 1/2 of a medium avocado, sliced
- 1 slice of whole-grain bread, toasted
- 2 tablespoons sprouts
- 2 tablespoons hummus
- ¼ teaspoon lemon zest
- ½ teaspoon hemp seeds
- ¼ teaspoon red pepper flakes

Directions:

• Spread hummus on one side of the toast and then top with avocado slices and sprouts. • Sprinkle with lemon zest, hemp seeds, and red pepper flakes, and then serve straight away.

Nutrition:

• Calories: 200 Cal Fat: 10.5 g Carbs: 22 g Protein: 7 g Fiber: 7 g

Apple and Honey Toast

Preparation Time: 5 minutes | Cooking Time: 0 minute |
Servings: 4

Ingredients:

- ½ of a small apple, cored, sliced
- 1 slice of whole-grain bread, toasted
- 1 tablespoon honey
- 2 tablespoons hummus
- 1/8 teaspoon cinnamon

Directions:

• Spread hummus on one side of the toast, top with apple slices and then drizzle with honey. • Sprinkle cinnamon on it and then serve straight away.

Nutrition:

• Calories: 212 Cal Fat: 7 g Carbs: 35 g Protein: 4 g Fiber: 5.5 g

Zucchini Pancakes

• Preparation Time: 10 minutes | Cooking Time: 15 minutes | Servings: 4

Ingredients:

- 2 cups zucchini
- 1/4 cup onion
- 1 tablespoon all-purpose white flour
- 1 teaspoon herb seasoning
- 1 egg 1 tablespoon olive oil
- 1/8 teaspoon salt

Directions:

• Grate onion and zucchini into a bowl and stir to combine. Place the zucchini mixture on a clean kitchen towel. Twist and squeeze out as much liquid as possible. Return to the bowl. • Mix flour, salt, and herb seasoning in a small bowl. Add egg and mix; stir into zucchini and

onion mixture. Form 4 patties.

• Heat oil over high heat in a large non-stick frying pan. Lower heat to medium and place
zucchini patties into the pan. Sauté until brown, turning once.

Nutrition:

- Calories 65, Total Fat 4.7g, Saturated Fat 0.9g, Cholesterol 41mg, Sodium 97mg, Total Carbohydrate 4.1g, Dietary Fiber 0.8g, Total Sugars 1.4g, Protein 2.3g, Calcium 16mg, Iron 1mg, Potassium 175mg, Phosphorus 24mg

Savory Spinach and Mushroom Crepes

• Preparation Time: 60 minutes | Cooking Time: 30-120 minutes | Servings: 4

Ingredients:

- For the crepes:
- 1 ¾ cup rolled oats
- 1 tsp pink Himalayan salt
- 1 ½ cup of soy milk
- 2 tbsp olive oil
- 1 tbsp almond butter
- ½ tsp nutmeg
- 2 tbsp egg replacement
- For the filling:
- 1 lb button mushrooms
- 10 oz fresh spinach, finely chopped
- 4 oz crumbled tofu
- 1 tbsp chia seeds
- 1 tbsp fresh rosemary, finely chopped
- 1 garlic clove, crushed
- 2 tbsp olive oil

Directions:

- First, prepare the crepes. Combine all dry ingredients

in a large bowl. Add milk, butter, nutmeg, olive oil, and egg replacement. Mix well with a hand mixer on high speed. Transfer to a food processor and process until completely smooth.

• Grease a large non-stick pancake pan with some oil. Pour 1 cup of the mixture into the pan and cook for one minute on each side.

• Plug your instant pot and press the _Sauté' button. Grease the stainless steel insert with some oil and add mushrooms. Cook for 5 minutes, stirring constantly.

• Now add spinach, tofu, rosemary, and garlic. Continue to cook for another 5 minutes.

• Remove the mixture from the pot and stir in chia seeds. Let it sit for 10 minutes.

• Meanwhile, grease a small baking pan with some oil and line with parchment paper.

• Divide the mushroom mixture between crepes and roll-up. Gently transfer to a prepared baking pan.

• Wrap the pan with aluminum foil and set aside.

• Pour 1 cup of water into your instant pot and set the steam rack. Put the pan on top and seal the lid. Press the _Manual' button and set the timer for 10 minutes.

• When done, release the pressure naturally, and open the lid.

- Optionally, sprinkle with some dried oregano before serving.

Nutrition:
- Calories:680, Total Fat:71.8g, Saturated Fat:20.9g, Total Carbs:10g, Dietary Fiber:7g, Sugar:2g, Protein:3g, Sodium:525mg

Spinach Pesto Pasta

• Preparation Time: 05 minutes | Cooking Time: 10 minutes | Servings: 2

Ingredients:

- 1cup pasta
- 2 cups spinach, chopped
- ¼ cup of coconut oil
- ½ large lemon
- ¼ teaspoon garlic powder
- 1/8 cup chopped pecans
- ¼ cup goat cheese, grated
- ¼ teaspoon salt
- Freshly cracked pepper to taste
- 2 oz. mozzarella (optional

Directions:

• Add the chopped and washed spinach to a food processor along with the coconut oil, 1/4 cup juice from the lemon, garlic powder, pecans, goat cheese, salt, and pepper. Purée the mixture until smooth and bright green. Add more oil if needed to allow the mixture to become a thick, smooth sauce. Taste the pesto and adjust the salt, pepper, or lemon juice to your liking. Set the pesto aside.

- Add pasta, water, and pesto, coconut oil into Instant Pot. Place lid on Instant Pot and lock into place to seal. Pressure Cook on High Pressure for 4 minutes. Use Quick Pressure Release.
- Add mozzarella cheese and serve.

Nutrition:
- Calories 534, Total Fat 35. 8g, Saturated Fat 27. 7g, Cholesterol 65mg, Sodium 514mg, Total Carbohydrate 39g, Dietary Fiber 1. 2g, Total Sugars 0. 7g, Protein 17. 5g

Paprika Pumpkin Pasta

• Preparation Time: 05 minutes | Cooking Time: 10 minutes | Servings: 2

Ingredients:

- ¼ cup of coconut oil
- ½ onion
- ½ tablespoon butter
- ½ teaspoon garlic
- ¼ teaspoon paprika
- 1 cup pumpkin purée

- 5 cups vegetable broth
- ¼ teaspoon salt
- Freshly cracked pepper
- 1 cup pasta
- 1/8 cup coconut cream
- 1/4 cup grated mozzarella cheese

Directions:

• Add the coconut oil to the Instant Pot, hit —Sautéll, Add butter and onion until it is soft and transparent. Add the garlic and paprika to the onion and sauté for about one minute more. Finally, add the pumpkin purée, vegetable broth, salt, and pepper to the Instant

Pot and stir until the ingredients are combined and smooth.

• Add pasta, then place a lid on the Instant Pot and lock it into place to seal. Pressure Cook on High Pressure for 4 minutes. Use Quick Pressure Release.

• Add coconut cream and mozzarella cheese.

Nutrition:

• Calories 327, Total Fat 8. 9g, Saturated Fat 4. 4g, Cholesterol 67mg. Sodium 931mg, Total Carbohydrate 49g, Dietary Fiber 4. 7g, Total Sugars 5. 7g, Protein 13. 5g

Creamy Mushroom Herb Pasta

• Preparation Time: 05 minutes | Cooking Time: 10 minutes | Servings: 2

Ingredients:

- ¼ cup of coconut oil
- ½ cup mushrooms
- ½ teaspoon garlic powder
- 1 1/2 tablespoon butter
- 1 1/2 tablespoon coconut flour
- 1 cup vegetable broth
- 1 sprig fresh thyme
- ½ teaspoon basil
- Salt and pepper to taste

Directions:

• Add the coconut oil to the Instant Pot, hit —Sautéll, add butter, when the butter melts add garlic powder, add the sliced mushrooms and continue to cook until the mushrooms have turned dark brown and all of the moisture they release has evaporated.

• Add the flour, Whisk the vegetable broth into the Instant Pot with the flour and mushrooms. Add the thyme, basil, and some freshly cracked pepper.

• Then add pasta, place the lid on the pot and lock it

into place to seal. Pressure Cook on High Pressure for 4 minutes. Use Quick Pressure Release.

• Serve and enjoy.

Nutrition:

• Calories 107, Total Fat 7. 5g, Saturated Fat 4. 8g, Cholesterol 15mg, Sodium 439mg, Total Carbohydrate 5. 7g, Dietary Fiber 2. 8g, Total Sugars 1. 3g, Protein 4. 2g

Cabbage and Noodles

• Preparation Time: 05 minutes | Cooking Time: 05 minutes | Servings: 2

Ingredients:

- 1 cup wide egg noodles
- 1 1/2 tablespoon butter
- 1small onion
- 1/2 head green cabbage, shredded
- Salt and pepper to taste

Directions:

• Add egg noodles, butter, water, onion, green cabbage, pepper, and salt to Instant Pot. Place lid on Instant Pot and lock into place to seal. Pressure Cook on High Pressure for 4 minutes. Use Quick Pressure Release.

• Serve and enjoy.

Nutrition:

• Calories183, Total Fat 6. 8g, Saturated Fat 3. 9g, Cholesterol 31mg, Sodium 78mg, Total Carbohydrate 27. 2g, Dietary Fiber 5. 9g, Total Sugars 7. 6g, Protein 5. 4g

Lemon Garlic Broccoli Macaroni

- 1 cup macaroni
- ½ cup broccoli
- 1 tablespoon butter
- ½ teaspoon garlic powder
- 1 lemon
- Salt and pepper to taste
- Enough water

Directions:

• Add macaroni, butter, water, broccoli, lemon, garlic powder, and salt to Instant Pot. Place the lid on the pot and lock it into place to seal. Pressure Cook on High Pressure for 4 minutes. Use Quick Pressure Release.

Nutrition:

• Calories 254, Total Fat 7. 4g, Saturated Fat 3. 9g, Cholesterol 62mg, Sodium 66mg, Total Carbohydrate 39. 8g, Dietary Fiber 1. 5g, Total Sugars 1. 3g, Protein 8. 4g

Basil Spaghetti Pasta

• Preparation Time: 05 minutes | Cooking Time: 05 minutes | Servings: 2

Ingredients:

- ½ teaspoon garlic powder
- 1 cup spaghetti
- 2 large eggs
- ¼ cup grated Parmesan cheese
- Freshly cracked pepper
- Salt and pepper to taste
- Handful fresh basil
- Enough water

Directions:

• In a medium bowl, whisk together the eggs, 1/2 cup of the Parmesan cheese, and a generous dose of freshly cracked pepper.

• Add spaghetti, water, basil, garlic powder, pepper, and salt to Instant Pot. Place lid on Instant Pot and lock into place to seal. Pressure Cook on High Pressure for 4 minutes. Use Quick Pressure Release.

• Pour the eggs and Parmesan mixture over the hot pasta.

Nutrition:

• Calories216, Total Fat 2. 3g, Saturated Fat 0. 7g, Cholesterol 49mg, Sodium 160mg, Total Carbohydrate 36g, Dietary Fiber 0. 1g, Total Sugars 0. 4g, Protein 12. 2g

Parsley Hummus Pasta

- ½ cup chickpeas
- 1/8 cup coconut oil
- ½ fresh lemon
- 1/8 cup tahini
- ½ teaspoon garlic powder
- 1/8 teaspoon cumin
- 1/4 teaspoon salt
- 1 green onion
- 1/8 bunch fresh parsley, or to taste
- 1 cup pasta
- Enough water

Directions:

- Drain the chickpeas and add them to a food processor along with the coconut oil, juice from the lemon, tahini, garlic powder, cumin, and salt. Pulse the ingredients, adding a small amount of water if needed to keep it moving, until the hummus is smooth.
- Slice the green onion (both white and green ends) and pull the parsley leaves from the stems. Add the green onion and parsley to the hummus in the food processor and process again until only small flecks of green remain. Taste the hummus and adjust the salt,

lemon, or garlic if needed.

• Add pasta, water into Instant Pot. Place the lid on the pot and lock it into place to seal. Pressure Cook on High Pressure for 4 minutes. Use Quick Pressure Release.

• In Sauté mode add hummus to pasta. When it mixes, turn off the switch of Instant Pot.

• Serve and enjoy.

Nutrition:

• Calories 582, Total Fat 26. 3g, Saturated Fat 13. 5g, Cholesterol 47mg, Sodium 338mg, Total Carbohydrate 71g, Dietary Fiber 10. 8g, Total Sugars 6. 1g, Protein 19. 9g

Creamy Spinach Artichoke Pasta

• Preparation Time: 05 minutes | Cooking Time: 05 minutes | Servings: 2

Ingredients:

- 1 tablespoon butter
- ¼ teaspoon garlic powder
- 1 cup vegetable broth
- 1 cup of coconut milk
- ¼ teaspoon salt
- Freshly cracked pepper
- ½ cup pasta
- 1/4 cup fresh baby spinach
- ½ cup quartered artichoke hearts
- 1/8 cup grated Parmesan cheese
- In the Instant Pot, hit —Sautéll, add butter when it melts, add garlic powder just until it's

tender and fragrant.

• Add the vegetable broth, coconut milk, salt, some freshly cracked pepper, and pasta. Place
the lid on the pot and lock it into place to seal.
Pressure Cook on High Pressure for 4
minutes. Use Quick Pressure Release.

- Add the spinach, a handful at a time, to the hot pasta and toss it in the pasta until it wilts into

  Instant Pot in Sauté mode. Stir the chopped artichoke hearts into the pasta. Sprinkle grated

  Parmesan over the pasta, then stir slightly to incorporate the Parmesan. Top with an

  additional Parmesan then serve.

Nutrition:

- Calories 457, Total Fat 36. 2g, Saturated Fat 29. 6g, Cholesterol 40mg, Sodium 779mg, Total Carbohydrate 27. 6g, Dietary Fiber 4g, Total Sugars 4. 7g, Protein 10. 3g

Easy Spinach Ricotta Pasta

• Preparation Time: 05 minutes | Cooking Time: 10 minutes | Servings: 2

Ingredients:

- ½ cup pasta
- 1 cup vegetable broth
- 1/2 lb. uncooked tagliatelle
- 1 tablespoon coconut oil
- ½ teaspoon garlic powder
- ¼ cup almond milk
- ½ cup whole milk ricotta
- 1/8 teaspoon salt
- Freshly cracked pepper
- ¼ cup chopped spinach

Directions:

• Add the vegetable broth, tagliatelle, spinach, salt, some freshly cracked pepper, and the pasta. Place lid on Instant Pot and lock into place to seal. Pressure Cook on High Pressure for 4 minutes. Use Quick Pressure Release.

• Prepare the ricotta sauce. Mince the garlic and add it to a large skillet with coconut oil. Cook over Medium-Low heat for 1-2 minutes, or just until soft and fragrant (but not browned). Add the almond milk and ricotta, then stir until relatively smooth (the ricotta may be slightly grainy). Allow the sauce to heat through and come to a low simmer. The sauce will thicken slightly as it simmers. Once it's thick enough to coat the spoon (3-5 minutes), season with salt and pepper.

• Add the cooked and drained pasta to the sauce and toss to coat. If the sauce becomes too thick or dry, add a small amount of the reserved pasta cooking water. Serve warm.

Nutrition:

• Calories277, Total Fat 18. 9g, Saturated Fat 15. 2g, Cholesterol 16mg, Sodium 191mg, Total

Roasted Red Pepper Pasta

- Preparation Time: 05 minutes | Cooking Time: 05 minutes | Servings: 2

Ingredients:

- 2 cups vegetable broth
- ½ cup spaghetti
- 1 small onion
- ½ teaspoon garlic minced
- ½ cup roasted red peppers
- ½ cup roasted diced tomatoes
- ¼ tablespoon dried mint
- 1/8 teaspoon crushed red pepper
- Freshly cracked black pepper
- ½ cup goat cheese

Directions:

- In an Instant Pot, combine the vegetable broth, onion, garlic, red pepper slices, diced tomatoes, mint, crushed red pepper, and some freshly cracked black pepper. Stir these ingredients to combine. Add spaghetti to the Instant Pot.
- Place lid on Instant Pot and lock into place to seal. Pressure Cook on High Pressure for 4 minutes. Use Quick Pressure Release.

• Divide the goat cheese into tablespoon-sized pieces, then add them to the Instant Pot. Stir the pasta until the cheese melts in and creates a smooth sauce. Serve hot.

Nutrition:

• Calories198, Total Fat 4. 9g, Saturated Fat 2. 2g, Cholesterol 31mg, Sodium 909mg, Total Carbohydrate 26. 8g, Dietary Fiber 1. 9g, Total Sugars 5. 6g, Protein 11. 9g

Cheese Beetroot Greens Macaroni

• Preparation Time: 05 minutes | Cooking Time: 05 minutes | Servings: 2

Ingredients:

- 1 tablespoon butter
- 1 clove garlic minced
- 1 cup button mushrooms
- ½ bunch beetroot greens
- ½ cup vegetable broth
- ½ cup macaroni
- ¼ teaspoon salt
- ½ cup grated Parmesan cheese
- Freshly cracked pepper
- In the Instant Pot, hit —Sautéll, add butter, garlic and slice the mushrooms. Add the beetroot

greens to the pot along with 1/2 cup vegetable broth. Stir the beetroot greens as it cooks until it is fully wilted.

• Add vegetable broth, macaroni, salt, and pepper. Place lid on Instant Pot and lock into place to seal.

Pressure Cook on High Pressure for 4 minutes. Use Quick Pressure Release. Add grated Parmesan cheese.

Nutrition:

• Calories 147, Total Fat 8g, Saturated Fat 4. 8g, Cholesterol 23mg, Sodium 590mg, Total Carbohydrate 12. 7g, Dietary Fiber 1g, Total Sugars 1. 5g, Protein 6. 5g

Pastalaya

• Preparation Time: 05 minutes | Cooking Time: 05 minutes | Servings: 2

Ingredients:

- ½ tablespoon avocado oil
- ½ teaspoon garlic powder
- 1 diced tomato
- ¼ teaspoon dried basil
- ¼ teaspoon smoked paprika
- ¼ teaspoon dried rosemary
- Freshly cracked pepper
- 1 cup vegetable broth
- ½ cup of water
- 1 cup orzo pasta
- 1 tablespoon coconut cream
- ½ bunch fresh coriander

Directions:

• In the Instant Pot, place the garlic powder and avocado oil, sauté for 15 seconds, or until the garlic is fragrant. Add diced tomatoes, basil, smoked paprika, rosemary, freshly cracked pepper, and orzo pasta to the Instant Pot. Finally, add the vegetable broth and ½ cup of water, and stir until everything is evenly combined.

• Place the lid on the Instant Pot, and bring the toggle switch into the —Sealing‖ position. Press Manual or Pressure Cook and adjust the time for 5 minutes.

• When the five minutes are up, do a Natural-release for 5 minutes and then move the toggle switch to —Venting‖ to release the rest of the pressure in the pot.

• Remove the lid. If the mixturelooks watery, press —Sauté‖ and bring the mixture up to a boil and let it boil for a few minutes. It will thicken as it boils. Add the coconut cream and leek to the Instant Pot, stir and let warm through for a few minutes.

• Serve and garnish with coriander toast. Enjoy!

Nutrition:

• Calories 351, Total Fat 6. 8g, Saturated Fat 3. 5g, Cholesterol 56mg. Sodium 869mg, Total

Pasta with Peppers

Preparation Time: 5 minutes | Cooking Time: 15 minutes | Servings: 2

Ingredients:
- 1 1/2 cups spaghetti sauce
- 1 cup vegetable broth
- ½ tablespoon dried Italian seasoning blend
- 1 cup bell pepper strips
- 1 cup dried pasta
- 1 cup shredded Romano cheese

Directions:

• Press the button Sauté. Set it for High, and set the time for 10 minutes.

• Mix the sauce, broth, and seasoning blend in an Instant Pot. Cook, turn off the Sauté

function; stir in the bell pepper strips and pasta. Lock the lid onto the pot.

• Press Pressure Cook on Max Pressure for 5 minutes with the Keep Warm setting off. • Use the Quick Release method to bring the pot pressure back to normal. Unlatch the lid and open the cooker. Stir in the shredded Romano cheese. Set the lid askew over the pot and set aside for 5 minutes to melt the cheese and let the pasta continue to absorb excess liquid. Serve by the big spoon.

Nutrition:
• Calories 291, Total Fat 6. 2g, Saturated Fat 2. 9g, Cholesterol 61mg, Sodium 994mg, Total Carbohydrate 43. 7g, Dietary Fiber 1g, Total Sugars 3. 5g, Protein 15. 1g

Lightning Source UK Ltd.
Milton Keynes UK
UKHW010652240621
386081UK00010B/559